HOW TO LIVE WITHOUT MEDICATION

50 COMMON HEALTH CONDITIONS THAT CAN BE RESOLVED NATURALLY

IRENE XANDERENA

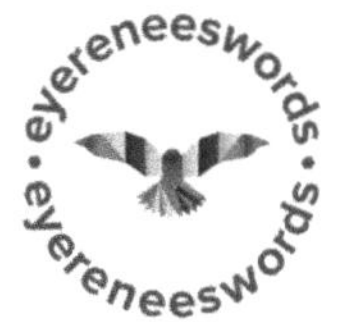

How to Live Without Medication

Copyright © 2023, Irene Xanderena

All Rights Reserved.

ISBN: 979-8-8689-3480-3

Published by

Eyereneeswords

Email: life@eyereneeswords.com

Website: www.eyereneeswords.com

Contents

Dedication

I dedicate this book to all the communities I have visited and had the privilege of serving during medical mission outreaches with Humanity First USA and The Xanderena Foundation.

Acknowledgment

I want to thank and acknowledge my mother, Mrs. Roseline Bosede Nwajei, and my aunty Mrs. Margaret Folake Araba, for teaching me about various herbs and the benefits of natural remedies. In this book, you will discover the importance of incorporating specific lifestyle habits. These beneficial practices encompass exercise, staying hydrated, consuming ample fruits and vegetables, opting for natural and unprocessed foods, prioritizing sufficient sleep, nurturing a positive mental state by reducing stress, and lastly, embracing the healing power of laughter.

Introduction

I started writing How to Live without Medication in 2018. My profession as a Registered Nurse exposed me to patients with acute and chronic health conditions, and 99% of the time, they were given one form of medicine or another.

Medicine involves using drugs, medical devices, and other therapies to help alleviate symptoms, cure diseases, and improve overall health. The goal of medicine is to improve the quality of life and extend the lifespan of the patient.

However, allopathic medicine, also known as Western Medicine, is the conventional or mainstream approach to healthcare. Allopathic medicine focuses on treating the symptoms of a disease or condition using medications, surgery, and other procedures. I witnessed many patients suffer through side effects, medication costs, and new symptoms resulting from their prescribed medication. You have probably seen commercials for different medications and a long list of identified side effects.

This book is a guide to using the homeopathic medicine approach. This is a form of alternative medicine that uses natural substances to treat a wide range of conditions. The basic principle of homeopathy is "like cures like," meaning that a substance that causes symptoms in a healthy person can treat similar symptoms in a sick person.

The benefits of using natural treatment include the following: fewer side effects, cost-effective, supports overall health, noninvasive, and sustainable. Homeopathic medicine aims to stimulate the body's natural healing processes to restore balance and health. Homeopathic medicine uses natural substances, such as herbs and minerals, in highly diluted forms to treat a wide range of conditions.

I was inspired to write this book when I volunteered with the Humanity First USA medical team in Guatemala and on many medical outreach missions in Nigeria, West Africa, with The Xanderena Foundation. Medication is expensive, and many members of the communities we visited cannot afford medicine. Many communities only receive medication when a medical outreach (such as ours) comes into their community for a day, and if they are fortunate enough, we give them free medication to last at least one month.

Preface

*"Let food be thy medicine and medicine
thy food."*
@ Hippocrates Asclepiades (460 BC – c. 370 BC.)
Known as the father of modern medicine.

I named this book 'How to Live without Medication" because it is a guide to Natural Medicine as a holistic approach to healthcare that utilizes natural remedies and therapies to prevent and treat illnesses. It is based on the principle that the body has an innate ability to heal itself and that natural remedies can support and enhance this process. Natural medicine includes a variety of practices, such as herbal medicine, acupuncture, massage therapy, chiropractic, homeopathy, and nutrition. These practices utilize natural substances, such as herbs, vitamins, minerals, and other nutrients, to promote health and wellness.

Natural medicine aims to treat the root cause of an illness rather than just addressing the symptoms. It also focuses on preventing illnesses by promoting healthy lifestyle habits like exercise, stress reduction, and a balanced diet. Natural medicine is in no way a quick fix! Hippocrates said, "Before you heal someone, ask him if he's willing to give up the things that made him sick." Living and maintaining a healthy life involves being an active participant in one's health.

Join me on this Homeopathic journey as you read "How to live without medication" As Hippocrates said, "The natural healing force within each of us is the greatest force in getting well."

Disclaimer

The information provided in this book is intended for educational purposes only and should not be considered a substitute for professional medical advice, diagnosis, or treatment.

Always seek the guidance of your healthcare provider or qualified practitioner before making any changes to your healthcare routine or embarking on any new treatment or therapy.

The content presented in this book is based on the author's research, personal experiences, and knowledge in the field of holistic care. However, individual experiences and responses to holistic practices may vary, and what works for one person may not work for another.

It is important to approach holistic care with an open mind, understanding that results may differ from person to person.

The author and publisher of this book are not liable for any direct or indirect damages or consequences arising from the use or misuse of the information provided.

Readers are encouraged to use their own discretion and judgment when implementing any suggestions or recommendations from this book. It is crucial to consult with a qualified healthcare professional or holistic practitioner for specific advice related to your individual health condition or concerns.

This book serves as a general guide and should not be considered a substitute for personalized, professional care. By reading this book, you acknowledge that you have read and understood this disclaimer, and you agree to assume all risks associated with the use of any information provided herein.

How to get rid of a headache naturally

1. **Drink water:** Dehydration is a common cause of headaches. Drink plenty of water throughout the day to stay hydrated and prevent headaches.

2. **Apply a cold compress:** Place a cold compress, such as a bag of frozen vegetables or an ice pack, on your forehead or neck to relieve pain and inflammation.

3. **Practice relaxation techniques:** Deep breathing, meditation, and yoga can help reduce stress and tension, which can trigger headaches.

4. **Get enough sleep:** Lack of sleep can cause headaches. Try to get seven to eight hours of sleep each night.

5. **Limit caffeine and alcohol:** Too much caffeine or alcohol can cause headaches. Limit your intake or avoid these substances altogether.

6. **Massage:** Gently massage your temples, neck, and shoulders to ease tension and promote relaxation.

7. **Use essential oils:** Peppermint, lavender, and eucalyptus essential oils may help relieve headaches. Apply a few drops to your temples or inhale the aroma.

8. **Eat a balanced diet:** Skipping meals or eating foods that trigger headaches can make them worse. Eat a balanced diet and avoid trigger foods.

9. **Exercise:** Regular exercise can help reduce stress and tension, which can trigger headaches. Try to get at least 30 minutes of exercise each day.

> **Comment**
>
> If your headaches are severe or persistent, it's important to see a doctor to rule out any underlying medical conditions.

TWO

How to reduce swelling in ankles naturally

1. **Elevate your legs:** Lie down and elevate your legs above the level of your heart to reduce swelling. This helps to improve blood flow and reduce fluid buildup in the ankles.

2. **Compression socks:** Compression socks can help improve circulation and reduce swelling in the ankles. They apply gentle pressure to the legs, which helps to promote blood flow and prevent fluid buildup.

3. **Exercise:** Regular exercise can help improve circulation and prevent fluid buildup in the ankles. Low-impact exercises such as walking, swimming, and cycling are recommended.

4. **Reduce salt intake:** Eating too much salt can cause fluid retention, leading to swelling in the ankles. Reduce your salt intake to help reduce swelling.

5. **Drink water:** Dehydration can cause fluid retention, leading to swelling in the ankles. Drink plenty of water throughout the day to stay hydrated and reduce swelling.

6. **Massage:** Gently massaging the ankles can help improve circulation and reduce swelling. Use your fingers to apply gentle pressure and massage in circular motions.

7. **Avoid standing or sitting for long periods:** Prolonged sitting or standing can cause fluid buildup in the ankles. Take regular breaks to move around and stretch your legs.

> **Comment:**
> If the swelling in your ankles persists or is accompanied by other symptoms, it's important to see a doctor to rule out any underlying medical conditions.

THREE

How to lose weight naturally

1. **Follow a healthy and balanced diet:** Include more fruits, vegetables, whole grains, and lean protein in your diet. Avoid processed foods, sugary drinks, and high-fat foods.

2. **Drink plenty of water:** Drinking water helps to flush out toxins and keeps you hydrated. It also helps to reduce hunger and can aid in weight loss.

3. **Exercise regularly:** Regular exercise is an excellent way to burn calories and lose weight. Even a little bit of exercise every day can make a big difference. You can start with simple activities like walking, cycling, or swimming.

4. **Get enough sleep:** Lack of sleep can disrupt your hormones and lead to weight gain. Aim for 7-8 hours of sleep and rest every night.

5. **Reduce stress:** Stress can lead to emotional eating, which can sabotage your weight loss efforts. Try to manage stress through meditation, yoga, or other relaxation techniques.

6. **Practice intermittent fasting:** Limit eating hours to occur within 10 hours a day. (Have your meals and beverages between 8 am to 6 pm). Practice having dinner between 5 pm to 6 pm. After dinner, avoid snacks and beverages with calories as this will spike insulin and prevent weight loss.

Comment:
It is always best to consult a doctor or nutritionist before making any significant changes in your diet or exercise routine. They can guide you on the best approach for your specific needs and health condition.

FOUR

How to reduce blood pressure naturally

1. **Lose weight:** Being overweight can contribute to high blood pressure. Even a slight weight loss can help reduce blood pressure.

2. **Exercise regularly:** Regular exercise can help lower blood pressure. Aim for at least 30 minutes of moderate-intensity exercise most days of the week.

3. **Follow a healthy diet:** A diet rich in fruits, vegetables, whole grains, and lean protein can help lower blood pressure. Avoid processed foods, high-fat foods, and foods high in sodium.

4. **Reduce salt intake:** Too much salt can raise blood pressure. Limit salt intake to less than 2,300 milligrams (mg) daily.

5. **Limit alcohol consumption:** Drinking too much alcohol can raise blood pressure. Men should limit alcohol intake to no more than two drinks a day, and women should limit intake to no more than one drink daily.

6. **Quit smoking:** Smoking can raise blood pressure. Quitting smoking can help lower blood pressure and reduce the risk of heart disease.

7. **Manage stress:** Stress can raise blood pressure. Try to manage stress through meditation, yoga, or other relaxation techniques.

Comment:

It is always best to consult a doctor before making significant changes in your lifestyle or treatment plan. They can guide you on the best approach for your specific needs and health condition.

FIVE

How to reduce anxiety naturally

1. **Exercise:** Regular exercise can help reduce anxiety by releasing endorphins and improving your mood. Aim for at least 30 minutes of moderate-intensity exercise most days of the week.

2. **Practice relaxation techniques:** Techniques such as deep breathing, progressive muscle relaxation, and meditation can help reduce anxiety and promote relaxation.

3. **Get enough sleep:** Lack of sleep can increase anxiety. Aim for at least 7-8 hours of sleep each night.

4. **Maintain a healthy diet:** A healthy diet can help reduce anxiety. Avoid processed foods, caffeine, and alcohol, which can increase anxiety.

5. **Limit exposure to stressors:** Avoid exposure to situations or people that increase anxiety. If you can't, learn coping strategies to manage stress when it arises.

6. **Seek social support:** Talking to friends or family members about your anxiety can help you feel less alone and more supported.

7. **Practice mindfulness:** Mindfulness involves being present in the moment and accepting your thoughts and feelings without judgment. This can help reduce anxiety and increase emotional awareness.

Comment:

It is important to seek professional help if your anxiety is severe or interfering with your daily life. A mental health professional can provide additional support and guidance.

SIX

How to get rid of heartburn naturally

1. **Avoid trigger foods:** Certain foods can trigger heartburn, including spicy, fatty, or acidic foods. Avoiding these foods can help reduce heartburn symptoms.
2. **Eat smaller meals:** Eating smaller meals throughout the day can reduce the amount of acid your stomach produces, which can help reduce heartburn.
3. **Stay upright after eating:** Lying down after eating can cause stomach acid to flow back into the esophagus, causing heartburn. Stay upright for at least 2-3 hours after eating.
4. **Wear loose-fitting clothing:** Tight clothing around the waist can increase pressure on the stomach, causing acid to flow back into the esophagus. Wear loose-fitting clothing to reduce pressure.
5. **Elevate the head of your bed:** Elevating the head of your bed by 6-8 inches can help prevent acid reflux while you sleep.
6. **Drink plenty of water:** Drinking water can help neutralize stomach acid and reduce heartburn symptoms.
7. **Try natural remedies:** Natural remedies like ginger, chamomile tea, and aloe vera juice can help reduce heartburn symptoms.

Comment:

It is important to seek professional help if your heartburn is severe or interfering with your daily life. A healthcare professional can provide additional support and guidance.

SEVEN

How to reduce abnormal bloating naturally

1. **Eat slowly:** Eating too quickly can cause you to swallow air, leading to bloating. Take your time to chew your food thoroughly and savor your meals.

2. **Avoid gas-producing foods:** Certain foods like beans, lentils, broccoli, onions, and carbonated drinks can cause gas and bloating. Avoid these foods if they cause bloating for you.

3. **Reduce salt intake:** Consuming too much salt can cause your body to retain water, leading to bloating. Try to reduce your salt intake, especially from processed and packaged foods.

4. **Stay hydrated:** Drinking plenty of water can help flush out excess salt and fluids from your body, reducing bloating.

5. **Exercise regularly:** Exercise can help move gas and fluids through your digestive system and reduce bloating. Try to get at least 30 minutes of exercise each day.

6. **Try probiotics:** Probiotics are good bacteria that live in your gut and can help improve digestion. You can get probiotics from fermented foods like yogurt, kefir, and sauerkraut.

7. **Manage stress:** Stress can affect your digestive system and cause bloating. Practice stress-reducing activities like deep breathing, meditation, or yoga.

> **Comment:**
> If your bloating persists or is accompanied by other symptoms, seeking professional help is vital. A healthcare professional can provide additional support and guidance.

EIGHT

How to get rid of bad breath naturally

1. **Brush and floss regularly:** Brush your teeth twice daily and floss once daily to remove food particles and bacteria that can cause bad breath.

2. **Use a tongue scraper:** Use a tongue scraper to remove any bacteria or debris on your tongue that may cause bad breath.

3. **Drink plenty of water:** Drinking water helps to wash away bacteria and food particles that can cause bad breath.

4. **Chew sugar-free gum or mints:** Chewing sugar-free gum or sucking on sugar-free mints can help stimulate saliva production, which can help to wash away bacteria and neutralize odors.

5. **Avoid foods that cause bad breath:** Certain foods like garlic, onions, and spicy foods can cause bad breath. Avoiding these foods can help reduce bad breath.

6. **Eat a healthy diet:** A healthy diet can help prevent bad breath by reducing the buildup of bacteria in your mouth.

7. **Practice good oral hygiene:** Besides brushing and flossing, mouthwash can also help kill bacteria that cause bad breath.

8. **Quit smoking:** Smoking can cause bad breath and increase your risk of gum disease. Quitting smoking can help to improve your breath and overall health.

Comment:

If your bad breath persists or is accompanied by other symptoms, it's important to seek professional help. A healthcare professional can provide additional support and guidance.

NINE

How to stop insomnia naturally

1. **Improve sleep hygiene:** Establish a regular sleep routine by going to bed and waking up at the same time every day. Avoid caffeine, nicotine, and alcohol before bedtime. Create a relaxing environment by keeping your bedroom cool, dark, and quiet.

2. **Limit screen time:** Screen exposure before bedtime can disrupt sleep. Avoid using electronic devices such as smartphones, tablets, and computers for at least an hour before bed.

3. **Practice relaxation techniques:** Relaxation techniques such as deep breathing, meditation, and yoga can help to reduce stress and promote relaxation, which can improve sleep.

4. **Exercise regularly:** Regular exercise can help improve sleep quality. However, avoid exercising too close to bedtime, as it can be stimulating.

5. **Avoid naps:** Taking naps during the day can interfere with your ability to sleep at night. If you do need to nap, limit it to 20-30 minutes and avoid napping in the late afternoon or evening.

6. **Use your bed only for sleep and sex:** Avoid using your bed for other activities such as reading, watching TV, or working.

7. **Try cognitive-behavioral therapy:** Cognitive-behavioral therapy (CBT) can help identify and change negative thoughts and behaviors contributing to insomnia.

8. **Consider natural remedies:** Some natural remedies, such as chamomile tea, lavender essential oil, and valerian root, may help to promote relaxation and improve sleep.

Comment:

If your insomnia persists or is accompanied by other symptoms, seeking professional help is important. A healthcare professional can provide additional support and guidance.

TEN

How to improve concentration naturally

1. **Create a distraction-free environment:** Minimize distractions by finding a quiet and comfortable place to work or study. Turn off your phone, close unnecessary tabs on your computer, and let others know you need uninterrupted time.

2. **Use the Pomodoro technique:** Break your work into 25-minute intervals, with short breaks in between. This can help you stay focused and avoid burnout.

3. **Stay organized:** Keep a to-do list and prioritize tasks. This can help you stay on track and avoid feeling overwhelmed.

4. **Take regular breaks:** Taking short breaks can help refresh your mind and improve productivity. Step away from your work and engage in a different activity to recharge your brain.

5. **Exercise regularly:** Exercise can improve blood flow to the brain and increase focus and concentration. Even a short walk or stretching can help.

6. **Eat a healthy diet:** Eating a balanced diet can help improve brain function and concentration. Avoid sugary or processed foods that can cause a crash in energy and focus.

7. **Get enough sleep:** Lack of sleep can affect concentration and productivity. Make sure to get enough restful sleep each night.

8. **Practice deep breathing:** Deep breathing exercises can help calm the mind and improve focus. Take a few deep breaths before starting work or when feeling distracted.

9. **Listen to music:** Listening to music can improve mood and focus. Choose music without lyrics or with a slow tempo to avoid distraction.

Comment:

Implementing these tips can improve your concentration and productivity without medication. However, if you continue to have difficulty with concentration, it may be helpful to seek professional help.

ELEVEN

How to reduce the risk of type 2 diabetes naturally.

1. **Maintain a healthy diet:** Eating a balanced diet with complex carbohydrates such as fruits, vegetables, whole grains, legumes, lean protein, and healthy fats can help manage blood sugar levels. Avoid simple carbohydrates such as sugary and processed foods.

2. **Exercise regularly:** Regular exercise can help improve insulin sensitivity and manage blood sugar levels. Aim for at least 30 minutes of moderate exercise most days of the week.

3. **Manage stress:** Stress can affect blood sugar levels, so it is essential to practice stress-management techniques such as deep breathing, yoga, or meditation.

4. **Get enough sleep:** Lack of sleep can affect blood sugar levels, so getting enough restful sleep each night is crucial.

5. **Monitor blood sugar levels:** Regularly monitoring blood sugar levels can help identify patterns and make necessary adjustments to diet and exercise.

6. **Lose weight:** Losing weight can help improve insulin sensitivity and manage blood sugar levels.

7. **Quit smoking:** Smoking can increase the risk of complications from diabetes, so it is important to quit smoking.

Comment:

It is important to note that medication may be necessary for some individuals with type 2 diabetes, and lifestyle changes may not be enough to manage blood sugar levels. Working with a healthcare provider to develop an individualized treatment plan is essential.

TWELVE

How to maintain a healthy colon naturally

1. **Eat a fiber-rich diet:** A fiber-rich diet can help promote regular bowel movements and reduce the risk of colon cancer. Good sources of fiber include fruits, vegetables, whole grains, nuts, and seeds.

2. **Stay hydrated:** Drinking plenty of water can help keep the colon hydrated and promote regular bowel movements.

3. **Exercise regularly:** Regular exercise can help promote regular bowel movements and reduce the risk of colon cancer.

4. **Limit alcohol and processed foods:** Consuming too much alcohol and processed foods can increase the risk of colon cancer.

5. **Get screened for colon cancer:** Regular age-appropriate colon cancer screening can help detect and treat colon cancer early.

6. **Don't smoke:** Smoking can increase the risk of colon cancer, so it is important to quit smoking.

7. **Manage stress:** Chronic stress can affect the digestive system and increase the risk of colon cancer. Managing stress through techniques such as deep breathing, yoga, or meditation can help promote a healthy colon.

8. **Get enough sleep:** Lack of sleep can affect the digestive system, so getting enough restful sleep each night is necessary.

9. **Practice good hygiene:** Practicing good hygiene, such as washing hands before eating and after using the bathroom, can help prevent the spread of harmful bacteria that can lead to colon problems.

> **Comment:**
> It is important to note that medication may be necessary for some individuals with colon problems, and lifestyle changes may not be enough to maintain colon health. Ensure you work with a healthcare provider to develop an individualized treatment plan.

THIRTEEN

How to stop diarrhea naturally

1. **Stay hydrated:** Diarrhea can cause dehydration, so it is important to drink plenty of water, clear broth, or other fluids to keep the body hydrated.

2. **Eat bland foods:** Eating bland foods like bananas, rice, applesauce, and toast (BRAT) can help ease diarrhea symptoms. Other bland foods like boiled potatoes and plain crackers can also be helpful.

3. **Avoid certain foods:** Avoid foods that can worsen diarrhea symptoms, such as spicy, fatty, or fried foods, dairy products, caffeine, and alcohol.

4. **Rest:** Resting can help the body recover from diarrhea and conserve energy.

5. **Use probiotics:** Probiotics are beneficial bacteria that can help restore the balance of bacteria in the gut. They can be found in foods like yogurt or taken in supplement form.

6. **Try herbal remedies:** Some herbal remedies, such as chamomile tea or ginger, can help soothe the digestive system and alleviate diarrhea symptoms.

7. **Use a heating pad:** Placing a heating pad on the stomach can help ease stomach pain and discomfort associated with diarrhea.

Comment:

It is important to note that if diarrhea persists for more than a few days or is accompanied by other symptoms such as fever or severe abdominal pain, individuals should seek medical attention as it may be a sign of a more severe condition.

FOURTEEN

How to stop constipation naturally

1. **Increase fiber intake:** Eating foods high in fiber, such as fruits, vegetables, whole grains, and legumes, can help soften stool and make it easier to pass.
2. **Drink plenty of water:** Staying hydrated by drinking water and other fluids can help soften stool and prevent constipation.
3. **Exercise regularly:** Regular physical activity can help stimulate bowel movements and prevent constipation.
4. **Increase magnesium intake:** Magnesium is a mineral that can help promote bowel movements. Foods high in magnesium include leafy greens, nuts, seeds, and whole grains.
5. **Use the bathroom when needed:** Ignoring the urge to have a bowel movement can lead to constipation.
6. **Try natural laxatives:** Certain foods, such as prunes, figs, and flaxseed, can act as natural laxatives and help promote bowel movements.
7. **Reduce stress:** Stress can contribute to constipation, so finding ways to manage stress, such as meditation, journaling, or yoga, can help prevent constipation.

Comment:

It is important to note that if constipation persists for more than a few days or is accompanied by other symptoms such as abdominal pain or bleeding, individuals should seek medical attention as it may be a sign of a more severe condition.

FIFTEEN

How to get rid of brain fog naturally

1. **Get enough sleep:** Lack of sleep can contribute to brain fog, so getting enough restful sleep is vital for mental clarity.

2. **Stay hydrated:** Dehydration can also lead to brain fog, so drinking enough water and other fluids like coconut water throughout the day can help keep the brain hydrated.

3. **Exercise regularly:** Exercise has been shown to improve cognitive function and reduce brain fog, so incorporating regular physical activity into your routine can be helpful.

4. **Practice stress reduction techniques:** Stress can contribute to brain fog, so finding ways to manage stress, such as meditation, deep breathing, or yoga, can be beneficial.

5. **Eat a healthy diet:** A diet rich in whole, nutrient-dense foods can help support brain function and reduce brain fog. Foods high in omega-3 fatty acids, such as nuts, and seeds, are particularly beneficial for brain health.

6. **Get outside:** Exposure to natural light and fresh air can help improve mental clarity and reduce brain fog.

7. **Engage in mental stimulation:** Challenging your brain with mentally stimulating activities, such as puzzles, reading, alternating using your dominant hand, or learning a new skill, can help improve cognitive function and reduce brain fog.

Comment:

It is important to note that if brain fog persists despite these efforts or is accompanied by other symptoms, individuals should seek medical attention as it may be a sign of an underlying medical condition.

SIXTEEN

How to get rid of indigestion naturally

1. **Avoid trigger foods:** Certain foods, like spicy or fatty foods, can trigger indigestion. Avoiding these trigger foods can help reduce symptoms.

2. **Eat smaller, more frequent meals:** Eating smaller meals throughout the day can help ease digestion and prevent indigestion.

3. **Chew food thoroughly:** Chewing food thoroughly and taking time to eat can help break down food more efficiently and reduce the risk of indigestion.

4. **Avoid eating close to bedtime:** Eating before bed can increase the risk of indigestion. It is recommended to avoid eating for at least 2-3 hours before going to bed.

5. **Drink plenty of water:** Drinking plenty of water and staying hydrated can help keep digestion moving smoothly and reduce the risk of indigestion.

6. **Avoid carbonated drinks:** Carbonated drinks can contribute to indigestion by causing gas and bloating. It is best to avoid these drinks or limit intake.

7. **Manage stress:** Stress can also contribute to indigestion. Finding ways to manage stress, such as meditation, deep breathing, or exercise, can help reduce symptoms.

8. **Try natural remedies:** Some natural remedies, such as ginger tea or chamomile tea, have been shown to help ease indigestion.

> **Comment:**
> It is important to note that if indigestion persists despite these efforts or is accompanied by other symptoms, individuals should seek medical attention as it may be a sign of an underlying medical condition.

SEVENTEEN

How to heal a sprained ankle naturally

1. **Rest:** Resting the injured ankle is crucial in allowing the tissues to heal. Avoid putting weight on the ankle and try to keep it elevated to reduce swelling. Use the RICE (Rest, Ice, Compression, and Elevation) therapy.

2. **Ice:** Applying ice to the ankle can help reduce swelling and pain. Apply an ice pack wrapped in a thin towel for 15-20 minutes at a time, several times a day.

3. **Compression:** Wrapping the ankle with an elastic bandage can help reduce swelling and provide support. Be careful not to wrap the bandage too tightly, restricting blood flow.

4. **Elevation:** Elevating the ankle above the heart can help reduce swelling. Keep the ankle elevated as much as possible, especially when resting.

5. **Exercise:** Once the swelling has gone down, gentle exercises can help improve flexibility and strength in the ankle. Consult with a healthcare provider or physical therapist for recommended exercises.

6. **Heat:** Applying heat to the ankle can help improve blood flow and reduce stiffness. Use a heating pad or warm towel for 10-15 minutes at a time, several times a day.

7. **Massage:** Gently massaging the ankle can help improve circulation and reduce stiffness. Use gentle pressure and circular motions to massage the ankle.

8. **Supportive shoes:** Wearing supportive shoes or using ankle braces can provide extra support and reduce the risk of re-injury.

> **Comment:**
>
> It is important to note that if the sprain is severe or does not improve with these measures, individuals should seek medical attention. A healthcare provider can provide additional treatment options and recommend physical therapy if necessary.

EIGHTEEN

How to stop a nosebleed naturally

1. **Pinch the nostrils:** Pinch the soft part of the nose (just below the bridge) with your thumb and index finger and apply gentle pressure for 10-15 minutes. This helps to compress the blood vessels and stop the bleeding.

2. **Lean forward:** Lean your head forward slightly to prevent blood from flowing down your throat. This can help reduce the risk of swallowing blood and vomiting.

3. **Apply ice:** Applying a cold pack or ice wrapped in a towel to the bridge of the nose can help constrict blood vessels and reduce swelling.

4. **Humidify the air:** Dry air can irritate the nose and cause bleeding. Use a humidifier or take a hot shower to add moisture to the air and soothe the nasal passages.

5. **Avoid blowing your nose:** Blowing your nose forcefully can irritate the nasal lining and cause bleeding. Try to avoid blowing your nose for a few hours after a nosebleed.

6. **Avoid hot and spicy foods:** Hot and spicy foods can increase blood flow and aggravate the nasal lining. Avoid such foods until the nosebleed stops.

Comment:

If the nosebleed does not stop after 20 minutes, or if you experience frequent nosebleeds, it is important to seek medical attention as it may be a sign of an underlying medical condition.

NINETEEN

How to maintain healthy eyes naturally

1. **Eat a healthy diet:** A diet rich in fruits, vegetables, and omega-3 fatty acids can help protect your eyes from age-related vision problems.

2. **Wear sunglasses:** UV rays can damage your eyes and increase the risk of cataracts and other eye problems. Wear sunglasses that block out 99% to 100% of both UVA and UVB radiation.

3. **Take breaks from the screen:** Staring at a computer, tablet, or smartphone screen for long periods can strain your eyes and cause dryness and fatigue. Take regular breaks at least every one to two hours to rest your eyes and reduce eye strain.

4. **Practice good hygiene:** Washing your hands frequently can help prevent eye infections. Avoid touching your eyes with dirty hands and avoid sharing towels or other personal items that may be contaminated.

5. **Exercise regularly:** Regular exercise can improve blood circulation and help maintain healthy eyes.

6. **Get enough sleep:** Lack of sleep can cause eye fatigue, dryness, and other vision problems. Aim for 7-8 hours of sleep per night.

7. **Visit your eye doctor regularly:** Regular eye exams can help detect vision problems early and prevent more severe eye conditions from developing.

> **Comment:**
> Following these tips can help maintain healthy eyes and reduce your risk of vision problems.

TWENTY

How to increase Oxytocin naturally

1. **Physical touch:** Oxytocin is often called the "cuddle hormone" because it is released when we engage in physical contact, such as hugging, cuddling, or holding hands.

2. **Positive social interactions:** Oxytocin is also released during positive social interactions, such as sharing a meal with friends or having a conversation with someone you care about.

3. **Meditation:** Studies have shown that meditation can increase oxytocin levels in the body.

4. **Massage:** Massage therapy has been shown to increase oxytocin levels and reduce stress.

5. **Laughter:** Laughter is a great way to boost oxytocin levels and promote feelings of happiness and well-being.

6. **Petting animals:** Interacting with animals, such as petting a dog or cat, can also increase oxytocin levels.

7. **Exercise:** Regular exercise has been shown to increase oxytocin levels and improve mood.

8. **Breastfeeding:** Oxytocin is released during breastfeeding and helps promote bonding between mother and child.

Comment:

By incorporating these natural methods into your daily routine, you can increase your body's production of Oxytocin and promote feelings of happiness, connection, and well-being.

TWENTY-ONE

How to increase serotonin naturally

1. **Sun exposure:** Exposure to sunlight can increase serotonin levels in the body. Spending time outdoors in the morning or early afternoon can be particularly helpful.

2. **Exercise:** Regular exercise has been shown to increase serotonin levels and improve mood.

3. **Eat a balanced diet:** A balanced diet that includes complex carbohydrates, such as whole grains, fruits, and vegetables, which can help increase serotonin levels.

4. **Tryptophan-rich foods:** Tryptophan is an amino acid that is a precursor to serotonin. Eating foods that are rich in tryptophan can help increase serotonin levels.

5. **Massage:** Massage therapy has been shown to increase serotonin levels and reduce stress. Getting a massage once or twice a month aids in serotonin promotion.

6. **Get enough sleep:** Getting enough sleep is vital for maintaining healthy serotonin levels. Aim to get 7-8 hours of sleep per night.

7. **Practice mindfulness:** Mindfulness practices like meditation, journaling, and yoga can help reduce stress and increase serotonin levels.

Comment:

By incorporating these natural methods into your daily routine, you can increase your body's production of serotonin and promote feelings of happiness, calmness, and well-being.

TWENTY-TWO

How to get rid of inflammation naturally

1. **Eat an anti-inflammatory diet:** Eating a diet rich in fruits, vegetables, whole grains, lean protein, and healthy fats can help reduce inflammation. Avoid processed foods, sugary drinks, and foods high in saturated and trans fats.

2. **Exercise regularly:** Regular exercise can help reduce inflammation. Aim for at least 30 minutes of moderate-intensity exercise most days of the week.

3. **Get enough sleep:** Getting enough sleep is vital for reducing inflammation. Aim for 7-8 hours of sleep per night.

4. **Manage stress:** Chronic stress can contribute to inflammation. Practice stress-reducing techniques such as meditation, yoga, or deep breathing exercises.

5. **Take omega-3 supplements:** Omega-3 fatty acids have anti-inflammatory properties and can help reduce inflammation.

6. **Use turmeric:** Turmeric contains curcumin, which has anti-inflammatory properties. Add turmeric to your food or take a turmeric supplement.

7. **Drink green tea:** Green tea contains polyphenols, which have anti-inflammatory effects. Drink 2-3 cups of caffeine-free green tea per day.

Comment:

By incorporating these natural methods into your daily routine, you can reduce inflammation and promote overall health and well-being.

TWENTY-THREE

How to reduce snoring naturally

1. **Change sleeping position:** Sleeping on your back can cause your tongue and soft palate to collapse to the back of your throat, obstructing airflow and causing snoring. Try sleeping on your side instead.

2. **Lose weight:** Excess weight can contribute to snoring by putting pressure on the airways. Losing weight can help reduce snoring.

3. **Avoid alcohol and sedatives:** Alcohol and sedatives relax the muscles in the throat, making snoring worse. Avoid consuming them before bedtime.

4. **Stay hydrated:** Dehydration can cause mucus to build up in the nose and throat, leading to snoring. Drink plenty of water throughout the day.

5. **Practice good sleep hygiene:** Establish a regular sleep routine and create a sleep-conducive environment. Keep the room cool, dark, and quiet.

6. **Use a humidifier:** Dry air can irritate the tissues in the throat, leading to snoring. Use a humidifier to add moisture to the air.

7. **Exercise regularly:** Regular exercise can help strengthen the muscles in the throat and reduce snoring.

Comment:

By incorporating these natural methods into your daily routine, you can reduce snoring and improve the quality of your sleep. However, if snoring persists or is accompanied by other symptoms, such as gasping for air during sleep, it is essential to consult a healthcare provider to rule out any underlying medical conditions.

TWENTY-FOUR

How to stop hiccups naturally

1. **Hold your breath:** Take a deep breath and hold it for as long as possible. This can help reset the diaphragm and stop hiccups.

2. **Sip cold water:** Take small sips of cold water slowly. The cold temperature can help relax the diaphragm and ease hiccups.

3. **Breathe into a paper bag:** Breathing into a paper bag can help increase the carbon dioxide levels in the body, which may help regulate the diaphragm and stop hiccups.

4. **Gargle with ice water:** Gargling with ice water can help stimulate the vagus nerve (also known as the tenth cranial nerve)which can help stop hiccups.

5. **Pull your knees to your chest:** Sit down and pull your knees to your chest, holding them there for a few minutes. This can help relax the diaphragm and stop hiccups.

6. **Swallow a teaspoon of sugar:** Swallowing a teaspoon of sugar can help stimulate the vagus nerve and stop hiccups.

7. **Breathe deeply:** Take slow, deep breaths and exhale slowly. This can help relax the diaphragm and ease hiccups.

Comment:

By trying these natural methods, you can stop hiccups without using medication. However, if hiccups persist or are accompanied by other symptoms, it is important to consult a healthcare provider to rule out any underlying medical conditions.

TWENTY-FIVE

How to prevent dehydration naturally

1. **Drink water:** The most effective way to get rid of dehydration is to drink water. Sip water slowly and continuously throughout the day rather than drinking large amounts at once.

2. **Eat hydrating foods:** Foods like fresh fruits and vegetables, soups, and broths can help replenish fluids and electrolytes in the body.

3. **Drink coconut water:** Coconut water is a natural electrolyte that can help replenish the fluids and electrolytes lost from the body.

4. **Drink sports drinks:** Sports drinks contain electrolytes that can help replenish fluids and electrolytes lost from the body during physical activity. Be sure to pick a natural sports drink with reduced simple sugar.

5. **Avoid caffeine and alcohol:** Caffeine and alcohol can dehydrate the body, so it is crucial to limit or avoid them when dehydrated.

6. **Rest:** Resting can help the body recover from dehydration, as the body can conserve fluids and energy.

7. **Use a cool compress:** Applying a cool compress to the skin can help cool the body and reduce the symptoms of dehydration.

Comment:

By trying these natural methods, you can eliminate dehydration without using medication. However, if dehydration persists or is accompanied by other symptoms, it is important to consult a healthcare provider to rule out any underlying medical conditions.

TWENTY-SIX

How to get rid of muscle pain naturally

1. **Rest:** Resting the affected muscle can help reduce pain and promote healing. Avoid activities that may aggravate the pain.
2. **Apply heat or cold:** Applying heat or cold to the affected area can help reduce pain and inflammation. Use a heating pad or warm towel for muscle soreness and a cold compress for acute injuries.
3. **Stretching:** Gentle stretching can help relieve muscle pain and promote flexibility. However, avoid stretching too vigorously, which can cause further injury.
4. **Massage:** Massaging the affected area can help promote blood flow and reduce muscle tension.
5. **Epsom salt bath:** Soaking in an Epsom salt bath can help relax muscles and reduce pain and inflammation.
6. **Stay hydrated:** Drinking plenty of water can help keep muscles hydrated and prevent cramping.
7. **Get enough sleep:** Getting enough sleep can help reduce muscle pain and promote healing.

Comment:

By trying these natural methods, you can get rid of muscle pain without using medication. However, if the pain persists or is accompanied by other symptoms, it is important to consult a healthcare provider to rule out any underlying medical conditions.

TWENTY-SEVEN

How to get rid of stomach cramps naturally

1. **Drink plenty of water:** Staying hydrated can help prevent and alleviate stomach cramps.

2. **Apply heat:** Applying heat to the affected area can help relax muscles and reduce pain. Try using a heating pad or a warm towel.

3. **Peppermint oil:** Peppermint oil has antispasmodic properties that can help relax muscles and reduce stomach cramps. Mix a few drops of peppermint oil with a carrier oil, such as coconut oil, and massage onto the stomach.

4. **Ginger:** Ginger has anti-inflammatory properties that can help reduce pain and inflammation in the stomach. Try drinking ginger tea or adding fresh ginger to meals.

5. **Chamomile tea:** Chamomile tea has anti-inflammatory and antispasmodic properties that can help alleviate stomach cramps. Drink chamomile tea to help soothe the stomach.

6. **Probiotics:** Probiotics can help restore the balance of good bacteria in the gut, which can help alleviate stomach cramps. Eat probiotic-rich foods, such as yogurt, kimchi, or sauerkraut.

7. **Avoid trigger foods:** Certain foods can trigger stomach cramps, such as spicy or fatty foods, dairy products,

and caffeine. Avoiding these foods can help prevent stomach cramps.

> **Comment:**
> By trying these natural remedies, you can help alleviate stomach cramps. However, if the pain persists or is accompanied by other symptoms, it is important to consult a healthcare provider to rule out any underlying medical conditions.

TWENTY-EIGHT

How to get rid of nail fungus naturally

1. **Tea tree oil:** Tea tree oil has antifungal properties that can help treat nail fungus. Mix a few drops of tea tree oil with a carrier oil, such as coconut oil, and apply it to the affected nail.

2. **Vinegar:** Vinegar has antifungal properties that can help treat nail fungus. Mix equal parts of vinegar and water and soak the affected nail in the solution for 15-20 minutes daily.

3. **Baking soda:** Baking soda has antifungal properties that can help treat nail fungus. Mix baking soda with water to form a paste and apply it to the affected nail. Let it sit for 10-15 minutes before rinsing it off.

4. **Garlic:** Garlic has antifungal properties that can help treat nail fungus. Crush a few garlic cloves and apply the paste to the affected nail. Cover it with a bandage and leave it on for a few hours before rinsing it off.

5. **Coconut oil:** Coconut oil has antifungal properties that can help treat nail fungus. Apply coconut oil to the affected nail and let it sit for a few hours before rinsing it off.

6. **Keep the affected area clean and dry:** Keeping the affected nail clean and dry can help prevent the growth and spread of nail fungus.

Comment:

By trying these natural remedies, you can help alleviate nail fungus. However, if the fungus persists or is accompanied by other symptoms, it is important to consult a healthcare provider to rule out any underlying medical conditions.

TWENTY-NINE

How to get rid of athlete's foot naturally

1. **Tea tree oil:** Tea tree oil has antifungal and antibacterial properties that can help treat athlete's foot. Mix a few drops of tea tree oil with a carrier oil, such as coconut oil, and apply it to the affected area.

2. **Vinegar:** Vinegar has antifungal properties that can help treat athlete's foot. Mix equal parts of vinegar and water and soak the affected foot in the solution for 15-20 minutes daily.

3. **Baking soda:** Baking soda can help reduce the itching and burning associated with athlete's foot. Mix baking soda with water to form a paste and apply it to the affected area. Let it sit for 10-15 minutes before rinsing it off.

4. **Garlic:** Garlic has antifungal and antibacterial properties that can help treat athlete's foot. Crush a few garlic cloves and apply the paste to the affected area. Cover it with a bandage and leave it on for a few hours before rinsing it off.

5. **Keep your feet clean and dry:** Keeping your feet clean and dry can help prevent the growth and spread of athlete's foot. Be sure to dry your feet thoroughly after showering or swimming.

6. **Wear breathable shoes and socks:** Wearing breathable shoes and socks can help prevent the buildup of moisture that can lead to athlete's foot.

> **Comment:**
> By trying these natural remedies and taking preventative measures, you can help alleviate athlete's foot. However, if the symptoms persist or worsen, it is essential to consult with a healthcare provider to rule out any underlying medical conditions.

THIRTY

How to get rid of jock itch naturally

1. **Tea tree oil:** Tea tree oil has antifungal and antibacterial properties that can help treat jock itch. Mix a few drops of tea tree oil with a carrier oil, such as coconut oil, and apply it to the affected area.

2. **Apple cider vinegar:** Apple cider vinegar has antifungal properties that can help treat jock itch. Mix equal parts of apple cider vinegar and water and apply it to the affected area using a cotton ball.

3. **Baking soda:** Baking soda can help reduce the itching and burning associated with jock itch. Mix baking soda with water to form a paste and apply it to the affected area. Let it sit for 10-15 minutes before rinsing it off.

4. **Coconut oil:** Coconut oil has antifungal properties that can help treat jock itch. Apply coconut oil directly to the affected area.

5. **Keep the affected area clean and dry:** Keeping the affected area clean and dry can help prevent the growth and spread of jock itch. Be sure to dry the area thoroughly after showering or swimming.

6. **Wear loose-fitting clothing:** Wearing loose-fitting clothing can help prevent the buildup of moisture and sweat that can lead to jock itch.

Comment:

By trying these natural remedies and taking preventative measures, you can help alleviate jock itch. However, if the symptoms persist or worsen, it is important to consult a healthcare provider to rule out any underlying medical conditions.

THIRTY-ONE

How to get rid of body odor naturally

1. **Shower or bathe daily:** Regular bathing helps to remove sweat and bacteria from your body.

2. **Use an antiperspirant or deodorant:** Antiperspirants reduce sweating, while deodorants mask the smell of sweat.

3. **Wear breathable clothing:** Choose clothing made from natural fibers like cotton or linen, which allow your skin to breathe.

4. **Wash your clothes regularly:** Dirty clothes can harbor bacteria and cause body odor.

5. **Eat a healthy diet:** Certain foods like spicy or greasy foods can worsen body odor, so try to eat a balanced diet with plenty of fruits and vegetables.

6. **Stay hydrated:** Drinking plenty of water helps flush toxins out of your body, reducing body odor.

7. **Use natural remedies:** Some natural remedies like baking soda, lemon juice, or apple cider vinegar can help to neutralize body odor.

Comment:

By trying these natural remedies and taking preventative measures, you can help alleviate body odor. However, if the symptoms persist or worsen, it is important to consult a healthcare provider to rule out any underlying medical conditions.

THIRTY-TWO

How to get rid of backache naturally

1. **Exercise regularly:** Regular exercise can help to strengthen your back muscles and prevent future back pain.
2. **Practice good posture:** Maintaining good posture can help prevent back pain by reducing the stress on your spine.
3. **Use heat or cold therapy:** Applying a heat pack or cold compress to your back can help relieve pain and reduce inflammation.
4. **Try massage therapy:** Massage therapy can help relax tight muscles and reduce pain.
5. **Practice yoga or stretching:** Yoga and stretching can help improve flexibility and reduce back pain.
6. **Use a supportive mattress:** A mattress that is too soft or too firm can cause back pain, so choose a mattress that provides adequate support for your back.
7. **Maintain a healthy weight:** Excess weight puts extra stress on your back, so maintaining a healthy weight can help prevent back pain.
8. **Stay hydrated:** Drinking plenty of water can help keep your joints and muscles hydrated, preventing back pain.

Comment:

By trying these natural remedies and taking preventative measures, you can help alleviate backache. However, if the symptoms persist or worsen, it is important to consult a healthcare provider to rule out any underlying medical conditions.

THIRTY-THREE

How to stop smoking naturally

1. **Set a quit date:** Choose a date to quit smoking and stick to it.

2. **Make a plan:** Create a plan to help you quit smoking, including coping strategies for dealing with cravings.

3. **Identify triggers:** Identify the situations, people, or emotions that trigger your urge to smoke and avoid them if possible.

4. **Use alternatives:** Find healthy alternatives to smoking, such as chewing gum, drinking water, or taking a walk when you feel the urge to smoke.

5. **Get support:** Seek support from family, friends, or a support group to help you stay motivated and accountable.

6. **Practice relaxation techniques:** Practice relaxation techniques such as deep breathing, meditation, or yoga to reduce stress and anxiety.

7. **Exercise regularly:** Exercise can help reduce cravings and improve your overall health.

8. **Keep yourself busy:** Engage in activities that keep you busy and distracted from smoking, such as reading a book, gardening, or painting.

9. **Reward yourself:** Reward yourself for reaching milestones in your journey to quit smoking, such as a massage or a special treat.

Comment:

Trying these natural remedies and taking preventative measures can help you stop smoking. However, if this void creates other concerns, consulting with a healthcare provider to rule out any underlying medical conditions is essential.

THIRTY-FOUR

How to stop coughing naturally

1. **Honey:** Honey has antibacterial properties that help soothe a cough. Mix a teaspoon of honey with warm water or herbal tea and drink it before bed.
2. **Ginger:** Ginger has anti-inflammatory properties that can help reduce coughing. Cut a piece of fresh ginger and boil it in water to make ginger tea.
3. **Saltwater gargle:** Mix a teaspoon of salt in warm water and gargle with it to soothe a sore throat and reduce coughing.
4. **Steam inhalation:** Inhaling steam can help reduce coughing and loosen mucus. Boil water and then hold your head over the pot with a towel covering your head to trap the steam.
5. **Eucalyptus oil:** Eucalyptus oil has antibacterial properties that can help reduce coughing. Add a few drops of eucalyptus oil to a bowl of hot water and inhale the steam.
6. **Thyme:** Thyme has antibacterial and antifungal properties that can help reduce coughing. Brew thyme tea by steeping fresh thyme in hot water for 10 minutes.
7. **Hydration:** Staying hydrated can help reduce coughing and soothe a sore throat. Drink plenty of water and herbal tea throughout the day.

Comment:

If your cough persists or is accompanied by other symptoms, it is important to consult with your healthcare provider.

THIRTY-FIVE

How to get rid of warts naturally

1. **Duct tape:** Cover the wart with duct tape for six days, then remove the tape and soak the wart in warm water. Use a pumice stone or emery board to gently remove dead skin, then repeat the process until the wart is gone.

2. **Apple cider vinegar:** Soak a cotton ball in apple cider vinegar and place it on the wart. Cover with a bandage and leave on overnight. Repeat nightly until the wart is gone.

3. **Garlic:** Crush a garlic clove and apply it to the wart. Cover with a bandage and leave on overnight. Repeat nightly until the wart is gone.

4. **Tea tree oil:** Apply tea tree oil to the wart with a cotton ball and cover with a bandage. Repeat twice daily until the wart is gone.

5. **Banana peel:** Rub the inside of a banana peel on the wart and cover with a bandage. Repeat nightly until the wart is gone.

6. **Aloe vera:** Apply aloe vera gel to the wart and cover with a bandage. Repeat twice daily until the wart is gone.

Comment:

These remedies may take several weeks or even months to work, and it is important to be patient and consistent with treatment. If the wart persists or is causing significant discomfort, it is important to consult with your healthcare provider.

THIRTY-SIX

How to increase heart rate naturally

1. **Exercise:** Exercise is a great way to increase heart rate naturally. It can be as simple as going for a walk or doing some light cardio exercises like jumping jacks or jogging in place.
2. **Caffeine:** Caffeine is a stimulant that can increase heart rate. Drinking a cup of coffee or tea can help increase heart rate naturally.
3. **Deep Breathing:** Deep breathing exercises can help increase heart rate by increasing oxygen intake. Take deep breaths in and out, and hold each breath for a few seconds before exhaling.
4. **Cold Water:** Drinking cold water or splashing cold water on the face can help increase heart rate naturally by stimulating the body's natural responses to cold.
5. **Stress:** Stress can increase the heart rate naturally. Try watching a scary movie or doing something that makes you nervous or anxious to increase your heart rate.
6. **Music:** Listening to fast-paced music can help increase heart rate naturally by stimulating the body's natural response to rhythm.
7. **Laughing:** Laughing can help increase heart rate naturally by stimulating the body's natural response to happiness and pleasure.

> **Comment:**
> It's important to note that an excessively high heart rate can be dangerous and should be monitored closely. If you have any concerns about your heart rate, it's best to consult a medical professional.

THIRTY-SEVEN

How to get rid of calluses (corn) naturally

1. **Soak in warm water:** Soak the affected area in warm water for 10-15 minutes to help soften the callus.
2. **Exfoliate with a pumice stone:** Gently rub a pumice stone over the callus to remove dead skin.
3. **Use Epsom salt:** Add Epsom salt to the warm water and soak the affected area for 10-15 minutes to help soften the callus.
4. **Apply apple cider vinegar:** Soak a cotton ball in apple cider vinegar and apply it to the callus. Leave it on for 10-15 minutes, then rinse with warm water.
5. **Apply aloe vera:** Apply fresh aloe vera gel to the callus and leave it on for 10-15 minutes. Rinse with warm water.
6. **Use a moisturizer:** Apply a moisturizer or petroleum jelly to the affected area to keep it soft and prevent further callus formation.

Comment:

Being patient and consistent with treatment is important, as calluses may take time to soften and reduce in size. If the callus is causing significant discomfort or pain, it is important to consult with your healthcare provider.

THIRTY-EIGHT

How to stop bug bite itch naturally

1. **Apply ice:** Apply an ice pack or a cold compress to the affected area for 10-15 minutes to reduce swelling and itchiness.
2. **Use essential oils:** Apply diluted essential oils such as tea tree, lavender, peppermint, or eucalyptus oil to the bite to reduce inflammation and itchiness.
3. **Apply honey:** Apply a small amount of honey to the bite to soothe the skin and reduce itchiness.
4. **Apply aloe vera:** Apply fresh aloe vera gel to the bite to reduce inflammation and itchiness.
5. **Use baking soda:** Mix baking soda with water to make a paste and apply it to the bite to reduce itchiness.
6. **Use oatmeal:** Mix oatmeal with water to make a paste and apply it to the bite to soothe the skin and reduce itchiness.
7. **Rub a banana peel:** Rub the inside of a banana peel on the bite to reduce inflammation and itchiness.

Comment:
If you experience severe symptoms such as difficulty breathing, swelling of the face or throat, or dizziness, seek medical attention immediately.

THIRTY-NINE

How to reduce the risk of high cholesterol and slow down abnormal lipid levels naturally

1. **Maintain a healthy weight:** Being overweight or obese can increase your risk of high cholesterol. Therefore, maintaining a healthy weight through a balanced diet and regular exercise can help reduce your risk.

2. **Eat a heart-healthy diet:** A diet high in saturated and trans fats can increase your cholesterol levels. Therefore, you should eat a diet rich in fruits, vegetables, whole grains, lean protein, and healthy fats from sources like nuts, seeds, and olive oil.

3. **Exercise regularly:** Regular physical activity can help increase your HDL (good) cholesterol levels and lower your LDL (bad) cholesterol levels. Aim for at least 30 minutes of moderate-intensity exercise most days of the week.

4. **Quit smoking:** Smoking can lower your HDL cholesterol levels and increase your risk of heart disease. Quitting smoking can help improve your cholesterol levels and overall health.

5. **Manage stress:** High stress levels can increase your cholesterol levels. Therefore, finding ways to manage stress, such as meditation, yoga, or deep breathing exercises, is important.

6. **Limit alcohol consumption:** Drinking too much alcohol can increase your triglyceride levels, contributing to high cholesterol. Therefore, limit your alcohol consumption to moderate levels (up to one drink per day for women and up to two drinks per day for men).

7. **Get enough sleep:** Lack of sleep can contribute to high cholesterol levels. Therefore, aim for at least 7-8 hours of sleep per night.

Comment:

It's important to note that lifestyle changes may not be enough for everyone to control their cholesterol levels. In some cases, medication may be necessary. Therefore, it's important to work with your healthcare provider to develop a personalized plan to manage your cholesterol levels.

FORTY

How to effectively reduce an elevated heart rate naturally

1. **Deep Breathing:** Deep breathing can help relax the body and slow down the heart rate. Take a deep breath, hold it for a few seconds, and then exhale slowly.

2. **Yoga or Meditation:** Yoga or meditation can help reduce stress and anxiety, which can contribute to an elevated heart rate. These practices can help calm the mind and relax the body.

3. **Exercise:** Exercise can help improve heart health and lower an elevated heart rate. Start with low-intensity exercises such as walking, swimming, or cycling, and gradually work your way up to more intense workouts.

4. **Drink Water:** Dehydration can cause an elevated heart rate. Drinking plenty of water can help keep you hydrated and lower your heart rate.

5. **Avoid Stimulants:** Stimulants such as caffeine, nicotine, and alcohol can increase the heart rate. Avoiding or limiting the intake of these substances can help lower an elevated heart rate.

6. **Get Enough Sleep:** Lack of sleep can increase stress and anxiety, which can contribute to an elevated heart rate. Aim for 7-8 hours of sleep per night to help lower your heart rate.

7. **Relaxation Techniques:** Techniques such as progressive muscle relaxation, guided imagery, or aromatherapy can help reduce stress and anxiety, which can contribute to an elevated heart rate.

> **Comment:**
> If an elevated heart rate persists or is accompanied by symptoms such as chest pain, shortness of breath, or dizziness, it's important to seek medical attention.

FORTY-ONE

How to get rid of a cold naturally

1. **Stay hydrated:** Drinking plenty of fluids, such as water, herbal tea, and clear broths, can help thin out mucus and relieve congestion.

2. **Rest:** Getting adequate rest can help your body fight off the cold and reduce the severity of symptoms.

3. **Steam:** Inhaling steam from a hot shower or bowl of hot water can help relieve nasal congestion and soothe the throat.

4. **Saltwater gargle:** Gargling with warm salt water can help soothe a sore throat and reduce inflammation.

5. **Honey:** Adding honey to tea or warm water can help soothe a sore throat and reduce coughing.

6. **Ginger:** Drinking ginger tea or using ginger in cooking can help reduce inflammation and relieve congestion.

7. **Vitamin C:** Eating foods high in vitamin C, such as citrus fruits, kiwi, and strawberries, can help boost the immune system and shorten the duration of a cold.

Comment:

It's important to note that these natural remedies may not completely cure a cold but can help alleviate symptoms and support the body's natural healing process. If you have any concerns or your symptoms persist or worsen, it's best to consult a medical professional.

FORTY-TWO

How to improve thyroid function naturally

1. **Eat a balanced diet:** Eating a diet rich in whole foods, lean protein, healthy fats, and complex carbohydrates can help support thyroid function.

2. **Increase iodine intake:** Iodine is an essential mineral for thyroid function, so consuming iodine-rich foods such as seaweed can help improve thyroid function.

3. **Reduce stress:** Chronic stress can negatively impact thyroid function, so practicing stress-reducing techniques such as meditation, yoga, or deep breathing can be helpful.

4. **Exercise:** Regular exercise can help improve thyroid function by boosting metabolism and reducing stress.

5. **Selenium:** Selenium is another essential mineral for thyroid function, so consuming selenium-rich foods such as Brazil nuts and sunflower seeds can be beneficial.

6. **Reduce inflammation:** Chronic inflammation can impair thyroid function, so consuming anti-inflammatory foods such as turmeric, ginger, and omega-3 fatty acids can be helpful.

7. **Avoid goitrogenic foods:** Goitrogens are compounds found in certain foods, such as cruciferous vegetables (broccoli, cauliflower, and kale), that can interfere with

thyroid function. Limiting the consumption of these foods may be helpful for some people.

> **Comment:**
> Note that these natural remedies may not completely cure thyroid disorders. So, you need to consult a medical professional for proper diagnosis and treatment.

FORTY-THREE

How to get rid of a fever naturally

1. **Rest:** Getting plenty of rest is vital for allowing your body to fight off the infection causing the fever.
2. **Stay hydrated:** Drinking plenty of fluids such as water, herbal tea, or broth can help prevent dehydration and promote healing.
3. **Cool compress:** Applying a cool, damp washcloth to your forehead, neck, and wrists can help lower your body temperature.
4. **Cool bath:** Taking a cool bath or shower can also help lower your body temperature and provide relief.
5. **Lemon and honey:** Squeezing fresh lemon juice into warm water and adding honey can help soothe a sore throat and promote hydration.
6. **Ginger:** Ginger has natural anti-inflammatory properties that can help reduce fever. Drinking ginger tea or adding fresh ginger to your meals can be beneficial.
7. **Turmeric:** Turmeric is another anti-inflammatory spice that can help reduce fever. Adding turmeric to your meals or drinking turmeric tea can be helpful.

Comment:

It's important to note that you should seek medical attention if your fever is high or persistent. These natural remedies can help provide some relief but are not a substitute for medical treatment.

FORTY-FOUR

How to increase potassium naturally

1. **Eat potassium-rich foods:** Some of the best natural sources of potassium include bananas, avocados, sweet potatoes, spinach, tomatoes, oranges, and yogurt.

2. **Drink coconut water:** Coconut water is a great natural source of potassium and electrolytes.

3. **Snack on nuts and seeds:** Nuts such as almonds, cashews, pistachios, and seeds such as pumpkin and sunflower seeds are high in potassium.

4. **Add beans and lentils to your diet:** Beans and lentils are high in potassium and a great source of fiber and protein.

5. **Eat more omega-3 fatty acids:** Walnuts, flaxseeds, chia seeds, hemp seeds, edamame, seaweed, and algae are high in omega-3 fatty acids.

6. **Use potassium-rich herbs and spices:** Herbs and spices such as parsley, basil, cinnamon, and turmeric are all high in potassium.

> **Comment:**
>
> It's important to note that if you have a potassium deficiency or are taking certain medications, you should speak with your healthcare provider before increasing your potassium intake.

FORTY-FIVE

How to maintain healthy kidneys naturally

1. **Stay hydrated:** Drinking plenty of water can help flush out toxins from the kidneys and keep them healthy.

2. **Eat a healthy diet:** Choose a diet rich in fruits, vegetables, whole grains, and lean protein. Your diet should also be low in sodium, sugar, and unhealthy fats.

3. **Manage blood sugar:** High blood sugar levels can damage the kidneys over time, so it is important to manage blood sugar levels if you have diabetes.

4. **Exercise regularly:** Regular exercise can help maintain healthy blood pressure levels and improve kidney function.

5. **Avoid smoking and excessive alcohol consumption:** Both smoking and excessive alcohol consumption can damage the kidneys over time, so it is important to avoid or limit these habits.

6. **Manage stress:** High stress levels can increase blood pressure and damage the kidneys. Practice stress-reducing activities such as meditation, yoga, or deep breathing exercises.

7. **Get enough sleep:** Adequate sleep is essential for overall health and can help maintain healthy kidneys.

> **Comment:**
> It's important to note that if you have pre-existing kidney problems or are at risk for kidney disease, you should speak to your healthcare provider before making any significant lifestyle changes.

FORTY-SIX

How to get rid of hot flashes during menopause naturally

1. **Dress in layers:** Wear lightweight clothes made of natural materials like cotton or linen. Dressing in layers will allow you to remove clothing as you start to feel hot.
2. **Keep cool:** Use a fan or an air conditioning unit to keep your room cool and well-ventilated.
3. **Stay hydrated:** Drink plenty of water to avoid dehydration, which can worsen hot flashes.
4. **Avoid triggers:** Certain things like spicy foods, caffeine, alcohol, and cigarettes can trigger hot flashes. Avoiding these triggers can reduce the frequency and intensity of hot flashes.
5. **Relaxation techniques:** Relaxation techniques like deep breathing, meditation, or yoga can help reduce stress and hot flashes.
6. **Exercise regularly:** Regular exercise can help reduce hot flashes and improve overall health.
7. **Herbal remedies:** Some herbs like black cohosh, red clover, and evening primrose oil have been shown to alleviate hot flashes in some women. However, it's important to speak to your healthcare provider before trying any herbal remedies.

Comment:

Note that while these natural remedies may help alleviate hot flashes, they may not work for everyone. If your hot flashes are severe or impacting your quality of life, talk to your healthcare provider about other treatment options.

FORTY-SEVEN

How to reduce stress naturally

1. **Exercise regularly:** Exercise is a great way to reduce stress and boost your mood. Try to get at least 30 minutes of exercise most days of the week.

2. **Practice relaxation techniques:** Deep breathing, meditation, and yoga can help relax your mind and body.

3. **Get enough sleep:** Lack of sleep can increase stress levels. Try to get at least 7-8 hours of sleep each night.

4. **Eat a healthy diet:** A balanced diet can help reduce stress and improve overall health.

5. **Spend time in nature:** Spending time in nature can help reduce stress and promote relaxation.

6. **Connect with others:** Social support can help reduce stress. Spend time with friends and family or join a support group.

7. **Set boundaries:** Learn to say no to requests that are not essential or will overburden you.

8. **Prioritize self-care:** Take time for yourself, do things you enjoy, and relax.

9. **Laugh:** Laughter can help reduce stress and boost your mood.

> **Comment:**
> Remember, it's important to find what works best for you to manage stress. If your stress levels are impacting your daily life, talk to a healthcare professional for further guidance and support.

FORTY-EIGHT

How to get rid of acid reflux naturally

1. **Change your diet:** Avoid trigger foods that can aggravate acid reflux, such as spicy foods, citrus fruits, tomatoes, caffeine, and alcohol.
2. **Eat smaller meals:** Eating smaller, more frequent meals can help reduce the acid in your stomach.
3. **Don't lie down after eating:** Wait at least 2-3 hours after eating before lying down or going to bed.
4. **Elevate your head when sleeping:** Use a pillow to elevate your head and upper body when sleeping to prevent acid from flowing back into your esophagus.
5. **Chew gum:** Chewing gum can stimulate saliva production, which can help neutralize stomach acid.
6. **Drink ginger tea:** Ginger has natural anti-inflammatory properties that can help reduce acid reflux symptoms.
7. **Lose weight:** Excess weight can put pressure on your stomach, leading to acid reflux. Losing weight can help reduce symptoms.
8. **Manage stress:** Stress can trigger acid reflux. Practice stress-reducing techniques such as meditation, deep breathing, or yoga.
9. **Avoid tight clothing:** Tight clothing can put pressure on your stomach, leading to acid reflux.

Comment:

Remember, talking to a healthcare professional is crucial if you experience frequent or severe acid reflux symptoms.

FORTY-NINE

How to get rid of seasonal allergies naturally

1. **Limit exposure to allergens:** Stay indoors when pollen counts are high, keep windows closed, and use an air conditioner with a HEPA filter to capture pollen and other allergens.
2. **Take a shower:** Taking a shower and washing your hair after being outdoors can help remove any pollen or allergens on your skin or hair.
3. **Use a saline nasal rinse:** Saline nasal rinses can help clear the nasal passages of allergens and irritants.
4. **Try a neti pot:** A neti pot is a device used to flush out the sinuses with a saline solution. It can help relieve congestion and reduce inflammation.
5. **Drink herbal tea:** Some herbal teas, such as chamomile, ginger, and peppermint, have natural anti-inflammatory and antihistamine properties that can help alleviate allergy symptoms.
6. **Eat an anti-inflammatory diet:** Foods rich in antioxidants and anti-inflammatory compounds, such as fruits, vegetables, whole grains, and nuts, can help reduce inflammation and boost the immune system.
7. **Avoid dairy products:** Cheese and cow's milk are known to increase mucus production and trigger allergies.

8. **Use essential oils:** Essential oils, such as eucalyptus, peppermint, and lavender, can help alleviate allergy symptoms when used in a diffuser or applied topically.

Comment:

Remember, while these natural methods can help alleviate seasonal allergies, they are not a substitute for medical treatment if you are experiencing severe symptoms or have a history of severe allergic reactions.

FIFTY

How to boost the immune system naturally

1. **Eat a healthy diet:** A balanced diet with plenty of fruits, vegetables, whole grains, and lean proteins provides the nutrients your immune system needs to function correctly.

2. **Get enough sleep:** Getting 7-9 hours of sleep per night helps your body produce cytokines, which are proteins that help fight infection and inflammation.

3. **Exercise regularly:** Regular physical activity helps improve circulation, which allows your immune system cells to move more freely throughout your body.

4. **Reduce stress:** Chronic stress can weaken the immune system. Practice stress-reducing techniques such as meditation, deep breathing, or yoga.

5. **Stay hydrated:** Drinking plenty of water helps flush toxins out of your body and keeps your immune system functioning properly.

6. **Avoid smoking and excessive alcohol consumption:** Smoking and excessive alcohol consumption can weaken the immune system.

7. **Get adequate vitamin D:** Vitamin D helps regulate the immune system. Exposure to sunlight is a natural way to get vitamin D, but you can also get it from foods such as almond milk, soybeans, chickpeas, and mushrooms.

8. **Use natural remedies:** Some natural remedies have immune-boosting properties, such as echinacea, elderberry, and garlic. However, it's important to talk to a healthcare professional before using any natural remedies.

> **Comment:**
> Remember, while these natural methods can help boost your immune system, they are not a substitute for medical treatment if you are sick.

Glossary

1. **Abdominal bloating** – A condition where the abdomen feels full, tight, or distended. It is accompanied by gas, burping, and abdominal discomfort.
2. **Acid reflux** – Also known as gastroesophageal reflux disease (GERD), is a condition in which stomach acid flows back into the esophagus.
3. **Anxiety** – A normal and natural response to stress, danger, or a perceived threat. It is a feeling of uneasiness, worry, or fear. It can be mild or severe.
4. **Athlete's foot** – Also known as tinea pedis, is a fungal infection that affects the skin on the feet.
5. **Backache** – Also known as back pain. It is a common condition affecting the back muscles, bones, and nerves.
6. **Bad breath** – Also known as halitosis. It is an unpleasant odor or smell that comes from a person's mouth.
7. **Blood pressure** – The force of blood pushing against the walls of the arteries as the heart pumps blood through the body. It is measured in millimeters of mercury (mmHg) and is expressed as two numbers, such as 120/80 mmHg.
8. **Body odor** – An unpleasant smell that can emanate from the body due to the bacteria on the skin.
9. **Brain fog** – A term used to describe a feeling of mental confusion, forgetfulness, and lack of mental clarity.

10. **Bug bite** – A skin reaction caused by the bite or sting of an insect or other arthropod, such as a mosquito, tick, bee, wasp, or spider.

11. **Calluses** – Thick, hardened areas of skin that develop due to repeated friction, pressure, or irritation. Often appear on hands, feet, or other body areas subject to repeated rubbing or pressure.

12. **Cold** – Also known as the common cold. It is a viral infection that affects the upper respiratory system, including the nose, throat, and sinuses.

13. **Colon** – Also known as the large intestine. It is part of the digestive system responsible for absorbing water and electrolytes from indigestible food matter, producing and storing feces, and eliminating waste from the body.

14. **Concentration** – The act of focusing one's attention or mental effort on a particular task or object.

15. **Constipation** – A condition characterized by infrequent bowel movements or difficulty passing stool.

16. **Cough** – A reflex action of the respiratory system that helps to clear the airways of mucus, irritants, and foreign particles.

17. **Dehydration** – A medical condition that occurs when the body loses more fluids than it takes on.

18. **Diabetes (type 2)** – A chronic medical condition that occurs when the body becomes resistant to insulin, or the pancreas does not produce enough insulin.

19. **Diarrhea** – A common digestive problem characterized by frequent, loose, and watery bowel movements.

20. **Elevated heart rate** – Also known as tachycardia. It is a condition where the heart beats faster than normal. It occurs when the heart rate exceeds 100 beats per minute at rest.

21. **Eyes health** – Refers to the overall well-being and function of the eyes, which are vital organs responsible for vision.

22. **Fever** – A temporary increase in the body's internal temperature, usually in response to an infection or illness.

23. **Headache** – A common condition characterized by pain or discomfort in the head or neck region.

24. **Heartburn** – A common condition that is characterized by a burning sensation in the chest and throat.

25. **Hiccups** – involuntary contractions of the diaphragm muscle that separates the chest cavity from the abdominal cavity and is responsible for breathing. When the diaphragm contracts involuntarily, it causes a sudden intake of breath, which is then interrupted by the closure of the vocal cords, resulting in the characteristic "hic" sound.

26. **High cholesterol** – A condition characterized by an increased level of cholesterol in the blood. Cholesterol is a fatty substance essential for the body's normal functioning.

27. **Hot flashes** – A sudden feeling of intense heat that can cause sweating, flushing, and a rapid heartbeat.

28. **Immune system** – A complex network of cells, tissues, and organs that work together to defend the body against harmful pathogens such as viruses, bacteria, and parasites.

29. **Indigestion** – Also known as dyspepsia. It is a digestive problem that occurs when the digestive system cannot break down food properly.

30. **Inflammation** – A natural response of the body's immune system to injury, infection, or irritation.

31. **Insomnia** – A sleep disorder characterized by difficulty falling or staying asleep or a lack of restful sleep despite having the opportunity to do so.

32. **Jock itch** – Also known as tinea cruris. It is a fungal infection of the skin in the groin area.

33. **Kidneys** – Vital organs in the body that play a crucial role in maintaining overall health. They are bean-shaped organs on either side of the spine, just below the ribcage.

34. **Low heart rate** – Also known as bradycardia. It is a condition characterized by a heart rate slower than normal. A normal heart rate for an adult is typically between 60 – 100 beats per minute.

35. **Muscle pain** – Also known as myalgia, is a common condition characterized by discomfort or pain in the muscles of the body.

36. **Nail fungus** – Also known as onychomycosis. It is a fungal infection that affects the nails, fingers, and toes. It can cause the nails to become brittle, discolored, thickened, and distorted in shape.

37. **Nosebleed** – Also known as epistaxis. It is a common condition that occurs when there is bleeding from the blood vessels in the lining of the nose.

38. **Oxytocin** – A hormone produced in the hypothalamus and released from the pituitary gland. It plays a role in a variety of psychological processes.

39. **Potassium** – A chemical element with the symbol K and atomic number 19. It is essential for plants, animals, and humans. It is a major electrolyte in the body.

40. **Seasonal allergies** – Also known as allergic rhinitis or hay fever. It is an allergic reaction to pollen from trees, grass, or weeds present in the air during certain seasons.

41. **Serotonin** – A neurotransmitter that is found in the central nervous system, digestive system, and blood platelets. It is essential in regulating mood, appetite, sleep, and physiological functions.

42. **Smoking** – The act of inhaling and exhaling the smoke produced by burning tobacco or other substances such as cannabis or herbs.

43. **Snoring** – A common condition characterized by the sound produced during sleep when airflow through the mouth and nose is partially obstructed.

44. **Sprain** – A type of injury that occurs when a ligament, which is a strong band of tissue that connects bones to other bones, is stretched or torn.

45. **Stomach cramps** – A painful, spasmodic contraction of the muscles in the stomach or intestine.

46. **Stress** – A physiological and psychological response to a perceived threat or demand. It is the body's natural reaction

to a perceived challenge or danger. It can trigger a fight-or-flight response that prepares the body for action.

47. **Swelling** – A condition characterized by an increase in size or volume of a body part due to accumulation of fluid or inflammation.

48. **Thyroid function** – The ability of the thyroid gland to produce and release hormones that regulate metabolism and control various bodily functions. The thyroid gland is an endocrine gland that produces hormones that regulate metabolism, growth development, and many other bodily functions.

49. **Warts** – Small rough, hard growths on the skin caused by the human papillomavirus (HPV). They are common and can appear anywhere on the body but are commonly found on the hands and feet.

50. **Weight** – A total mass or weight of a person's body, including all tissues, organs, and fluids. It is typically measured in kilograms or pounds.

Bibliography

1. "Dr. Sebi's Cookbook: A Complete Guide to a Plant-Based Diet with 77 Simple, Delicious, and Easy-to-Make Recipes for Holistic Healing and Longevity" by Carin C. Hendry.
2. "Forks Over Knives: The Plant-Based Way to Health" by Gene Stone and T. Colin Campbell, Ph.D.
3. "How Not to Die: Discover the Foods Scientifically Proven to Prevent and Reverse Disease" by Michael Greger, MD.
4. "In Defense of Food" by Michael Polla
5. "Nutrition and Physical Degeneration" by Weston A. Price
6. "Plant-Based Nutrition, 2E (Idiot's Guides)" by Julieanna Hever, MS, RD, CPT.
7. "The 4-Hour Body: An Uncommon Guide to Rapid Fat-Loss, Incredible Sex, and Becoming Superhuman" by Timothy Ferriss
8. "The Alchemist" by Paulo Coelho
9. "The China Study: The Most Comprehensive Study of Nutrition Ever Conducted and the Startling Implications for Diet, Weight Loss, and Long-Term Health" by T. Colin Campbell and Thomas M. Campbell II
10. "The Complete Guide to Crystal Chakra Healing" by Philip Permutt
11. "The Encyclopedia of Natural Medicine" by Michael T. Murray and Joseph Pizzorno
12. "The Green Pharmacy" by James A. Duke
13. "The Healing Power of Essential Oils" by Eric Zielinski

14. "The Healing Power of Mindfulness" by Jon Kabat-Zinn
15. "The Healthy Mind Toolkit: Simple Strategies to Get Out of Your Own Way and Enjoy Your Life" by Alice Boyes
16. "The Plant Paradox: The Hidden Dangers in "Healthy" Foods That Cause Disease and Weight Gain" by Steven R. Gundry
17. "The Plant-Based Solution: America's Healthy Heart Doc's Plan to Power Your Health" by Joel K. Kahn, MD.
18. "The Power of Now: A Guide to Spiritual Enlightenment" by Eckhart Tolle
19. "The Tao of Health, Sex, and Longevity: A Modern Practical Guide to the Ancient Way" by Daniel Reid
20. . "The Omnivore's Dilemma" by Michael Polla
21. "Dr. Sebi Bible–The Ultimate Guide to a disease-free life. Everything you ever need to know about Dr. Sebi's Alkaline Diet, Herb selection, treatments, and cures for any diseases" by Serena Brown
22. Herbal Medicine: From the Heart of the Earth" by Sharol Tilgner
23. The Complete Book of Ayurvedic Home Remedies" by Vasant Lad